Carnivore Diet

A Complete Animal Based Diet For Strength, Energy, And Weight Loss Made Easy

Introduction

"To say that the oldest form of food is causing modern diseases ... is the most ludicrous thing I have ever heard" – Anonymous

Did you know that our ancestors adhered to a strict animal-based diet? Yes, long before the first humans realized they could start relying on wild fruits and practicing crop farming, meat was their primary source of nutrition!

And do you know what they got from relying primarily on meats for survival? Simple; long, healthy life where they are lean, agile, tall and free from the diseases of modern day life! The Maasai of East Africa along with many other communities around the world can attest to the goodness of the carnivore diet. It is only until recently that the vast majority of human race has started connecting the dots between the carnivore diet and long and healthy life! For years, the food pyramid hid us under a mountain of carbs, bread and industrialized modern seed oils. This is about to end, as more people realize that meats are not the enemy!

As controversial as it may sound about eating nothing else but animal related products, this ancestral diet will supercharge your health by improving your mental clarity, reduce bloating, kick start weight loss and give you a jolt of energy every day.

And lucky for you, this book will take you by the hand to help you adopt the diet with ease to start enjoying its many benefits!

Are you ready to get started? If you are, let's begin!

Thanks again for purchasing this book. I hope you enjoy it!

Table of Contents

If this is your first encounter with the term carnivore diet, you would be excused if you have questions about some of the basic things about the diet. That's why we will start from the very beginning i.e. building our understanding of what the diet is all about, its benefits, how it works, and more!

The Carnivore Diet: The Basics

What Is It?

The carnivore diet is a high protein and high fat diet where you only eat all kinds of meat, dairy and eggs while avoiding all plant based foods, including vegetables, fruits, seeds, nuts, grains and legumes – especially no carbs.

Some even recommend prohibiting or cutting down on dairy products that are low in lactose such as hard cheese and butter. Some strict proponents of the carnivore diet cannot even cook with olive oil or eat candy bars.

When you think of it, this is almost the complete opposite of a vegan diet, which teaches proponents to follow a strict, plant-based diet.

Basically, the carnivore diet boils down to one simple equation: Carnivore diet = meat + water.

It is that simple! In fact, the carnivore diet is one of the simplest and most straightforward diets because it does not provide any precise guiding principles with regards to how may meals or snacks to eat per day, the amount of serving sizes or the number of calories to take.

You eat as often and as much as you desire!

It works with weight loss because you really can't eat much owing to the fact that meat is very satiating and takes time to digest, which means it will take some time to digest. As a result, you can afford to go for a longer period without eating, something which will ultimately lower your overall calorie intake per day, create the needed calorie deficit for weight loss and much more!

Moreover, adopting the carnivore diet means freedom. Freedom from baking, meal planning, vegetable preparation, and you will wash up less.

The Carnivore diet as a sustainable way of eating

It is indeed possible for one to survive on an all meat diet since animal-based foods contain all the essential nutrients your body could need including, vitamins, amino acids, fatty acids (docosahexaenoic acid (DHA) and arachidonic acid (AA) and minerals.

The basic facts about human nutrition and biology show that the carnivore diet can be a sustainable way of living.

A good example is a clinical study that was conducted in 1928. Two men namely Anderson and Stefansson in New York's Bellevue Hospital ate nothing else for two years straight but an all-meat diet. After the two year experiment, tests showed that they were perfectly healthy, if not even more so.

Need more proof? Look no further than the hunter and gatherer communities such as the Maasai of East Africa and the Alaskan Inuit who live largely on highly carnivorous diets with pretty nearly no chronic diseases as compared to what we have in the Western world.

For a healthy human brain to grow and function it requires a large amount of energy and very specific quantities of nutrients that can only come by eating animal based foods predominantly. Such nutrients are the essential fatty acids (AA and DHA), minerals like selenium, zinc, iodine and iron; vitamins B, D, A (and especially vitamin B12 which cannot be found in plant based foods). Based on some research studies, it is believed that if it weren't for meat, the early men would never have been able to evolve with the brains we did. This is one of the reasons why even with all kinds of supplements, vegetarians have to be very careful if they need to provide their brains with all the essential nutrients that are needed.

Next, we'll discuss how the diet works to bring about the benefits.

How Does The Canivore Diet Work?

The carnivore diet and the ketogenic diet are similar in that they both are high protein, high fat and low carb diets. When your body receives little or no carbohydrates for a long period of time, it shifts into a metabolic state known as ketosis.

Ketosis is a process in which the liver breaks down fat through oxidation to form ketones (a form of energy molecules) such as Beta-Hydroxybutyrate (BHB) and Acetoacetate. Fat is only broken down when there is a deficiency of glucose in the bloodstream. The ketones produced are an alternative source of energy when glucose is absent.

When the intake of carbohydrates is limited, the level of insulin drops substantially and this also leads to increased breakdown of fats. Ketones are then generated and they can be used by any cell or tissue in the body.

When you follow the carnivore diet strictly, your body switches almost entirely to run on ketones produced from fat. And since the body organs and in particular the brain requires a lot of energy to function, the diet should include a lot of fats.

Ketones are also considered to be more stable than glucose and therefore more efficient in providing more energy to the body cells. As a matter of fact, ketones have an approximate caloric value of 4.5 to 5.5 calories per gram; which is more than the energy produced by carbohydrates and proteins. Unlike glucose, ketone bodies do not rely on insulin to get in the cells. This means they don't pose any danger to your blood sugar regulation mechanism, which, if it is not working properly, can result to development of diseases like diabetes and various other metabolic disorders like heart disease.

Let's take this further where we discuss what's wrong with plant-based foods that we've been told for years are natures gift for our health!

Why Plants Don't Exist To Be Eaten

Should you eat meat or plants? This is usually a highly debated topic but we'll save that for another day. However, there are several reasons why vegetables and fruits are a no-go zone.

We all know that fruits contain a lot of sugar. Vegetables on the other hand carry a lot of starches. But that is not the point here. The main reason you should avoid plant based diets is because of their anti-nutrients.

What Are Anti-Nutrients?

For hundreds of millions of years, plants, just like any other living organisms, have fought for generation after generation to survive. Since plants cannot flee or fight from predators, insects and fungi, they developed clever mechanisms over millions of years of evolution to survive. They use defenses like thorns, spines and sharp prickles on their leaves and stems.

But as if that's not enough, plants use a cleverer and sophisticated arsenal of chemical weapons (anti-nutrients) to defend themselves. Some of these chemicals work by interfering with the predator's metabolism, others kill the cell's mitochondria and others launch an attack on the predator's DNA directly.

And it isn't only a few plants with such phytochemicals but all of them. Every variety and species of plants has its own unique set of anti-nutrients. Even the different parts of a plant have different anti-nutrients in varying amounts as explained below:

Salicylates - found mostly in pickles, cucumbers, coffee, cherries, berries, apricots, apples, almonds. Cause allergy like symptoms such as GI upset, constriction of bronchial passages, disturbed vision, headaches, restless leg syndrome and acne

Cyanogenic glycosides - Plants use it to kill insects and is found in over 2500 plant species including cassava and a number of fruits e.g. cherries and peaches. It causes goiter and hypothyroidism.

Photosensitizers - plant defense mechanisms that make predators sensitive to light (photodermatitis). Plants such as grapefruit, celery and lime cause swelling when you make contact with them out in the sun.

Flavonoids - found in soybeans and many fruits, Flavonoids can disrupt hormone function and cause estrogen like effects.

Sulforaphane - a pungent molecule found mostly in broccoli and other cruciferous veggies used to kill insects, fungi and bacteria. In humans, it causes cell death or damage to intracellular structures like mitochondria.

Glycoalkaloids - solanine and chaconine are both glycoalkaloids and large amounts are found mostly in potatoes though other nightshades such as tomatoes, peppers and eggplants contain trace amounts. Consumption of glycoalkaloids causes restlessness, insomnia, anxiety, diarrhea, vomiting and nausea. Severe cases include respiratory arrest, convulsions and paralysis.

Saponins - mostly come from soybeans. They help protect plants from fungi and microbes. They're resistant to digestion and cause leaky gut, inflammation and autoimmune diseases. Soy is also rich in other anti-nutrients such as trypsin, tannin and phytic acid.

Protease - are enzyme inhibitors mostly found in wheat and they interfere and block the digestion of protein.

Lectins - heavy concentrations are usually found in the seeds like beans, grains and nuts and even some fruits. The plant's intention is to protect the offspring from getting eaten by predators and thus the use of lectin. When consumed, lectins can cause agglutination, endocrine and cellular disruption, conditions that stem from autoimmunity (such as celiac's disease, lupus, crohn's disease etc), inflammation and leaky gut.

This list of secondary meatabloites only covers just a portion of the major players that have been studied and found to be harmful to humans. However, these are just a tip of the iceberg. There are literally tens and hundreds of thousands of these harmful bioactive compounds produced by plants; all the more reason why you need to stick to a carnivore diet.

So what will you be eating when you are following a carnivore diet? Let's discuss that next.

Carnivore Diet Food List

Below is a list of all the kinds of foods you can eat on a carnivore diet. Anything other than what is mentioned below is strictly prohibited.

Meat

Your main source of calorie should be acquired from all kinds of grass fed meat e.g. beef, lamb, goat and pork. You should especially go for the fatty cuts like the flank steak, pork chops, bacon, t-bone, 80/20 ground beef, ribeye, porterhouse and strip steak.

Since the carnivore diet restricts carbs, make sure you consume such meat with high fat content so that your body can use the fat as fuel.

If you fail to consume enough fats, you could develop *‘rabbit starvation’,* which is characterized by diarrhea, lethargy and headaches.

This condition develops when you try to subsist only on lean meat, which primarily comprises of protein without getting sufficient calories from either fat or carbs.

Poultry

This category includes chicken, duck, turkey, pigeons, geese and guineas etc.

Eggs

Popularly known as nature's multivitamin, eggs provide you with the perfect ratio of fats, proteins and other essential nutrients.

Fish and other edible aquatic animals

Just like meat, go for the fattiest fish such as tuna, mackerel, redfish, halibut, sole, codfish, herring, salmon, catfish, pike perch, whitefish, trout eel and carp among others.

There are also crustaceans such as jellyfish, octopuses, squids, mollusks, mussels, oysters, clams, mollusks, prawns, shrimps, crabs and lobsters.

Offal / Organ meat

This is a list of some of the edible organs of an animal that you can prepare for food: caul fat, oxtail, brain, sweetbreads (thymus glands), tripe, tongue, beef cheek, heart, kidney, liver, gizzard, pig's snout, lungs, roe (fish eggs especially from sturgeon or salmon), bone marrow, pork trotter and pancreas. Tallow, lard, schmaltz and other animal-based fats can be used to cook your food instead of using vegetable oil.

Dairy

This category is made up of foods that are produced from milk e.g. cheese, butter and cream. However, most of these contain carbs and most people on the carnivore diet tend to limit their intake or avoid them altogether.

Condiments

These include salt, pepper, spices, hot sauces and herbs to season and improve flavor to your meat. They are used in small amounts and their effects should be negligible. However, you need to be extra careful with these as some may contain carbs or sugars. You shouldn't use these if you have strong autoimmune sensitivities to plant compounds.

So after you've adapted a meat-based diet, what benefits should you expect from that? Let's discuss some of the science-backed benefits that come with following a carnivore diet.

Benefits Of The Carnivore Diet

1. Improved brain function and mental clarity

Anthropology studies show that our ancestors' transition from a plant based diet to a carnivorous one coincided with a massive expansion in the size of their brains. This alone is enough to show you how beneficial meat based diets are to your brain over time.

Moreover, many carnivores have reported reduced brain fog, improved mental clarity, energy and focus and a sense of calm that couldn't be attained when eating carbs.

The explanation to this could be that restricting carbs makes you fat adapted i.e. your body runs on ketones for energy. And studies show that ketone bodies posses neuroprotective properties and that the human brain prefers to run on fat rather than glucose for energy.

2. Supports weight loss

If the carnivore diet you follow is well designed to induce ketosis, then it will definitely enable you to lose weight. Ketosis promotes weight loss by increasing the metabolism of body fat. According to some studies, low carb diets suppress the production of insulin and in turn fat storage is prevented and weight loss is promoted.

Additionally, consuming plenty of protein and fat promotes satiety for longer. Once you fill up on fatty meaty, you won't be craving for snacks and it will take some time before you get hungry again. This means you end up consuming fewer calories. Moreover, a high protein diet enhances your body composition by making your body leaner.

3. Increased libido and testosterone

According to different studies, consuming **fresh** and **unprocessed** meat results in a decline in SHBG (Sex Hormone Binding Globulin), which translates to an increase in testosterone and the subsequent libido. However, this only applies to unprocessed meat. Actually, processed meats can greatly lower your testosterone levels.

Obese and overweight people are also likely to suffer from sexual dysfunction. If the carnivore diet can help you shed off a few pounds, then it will definitely restore sexual function.

Finally, consuming animal fats has been linked with restoring optimum hormonal function, including testosterone. The carnivore diet can therefore improve testosterone.

4.   Eliminates inflammation and food sensitivity triggers

You can improve inflammatory conditions such as Hashimoto and Arthritis by switching to a carnivore diet. Potentially inflammatory compounds such as histamine, lectins, oxalates and gluten are found in plant based foods. And this can cause serious illnesses especially if you are sensitive to such foods. However, switching to a carnivore diet decreases inflammation and makes you feel more energetic and healthier.

5.   Promotes growth and development

Animal-based foods such as meat, fish, milk and chicken are densely packed with nutrients such as protein, B vitamins, calcium and iron. These nutrients promote healthy growth and development especially for the teenagers and children. In one particular study, more than 3000 children and babies in the United States living in low-income families were fed with adequate meat consumption and it prevented stunting. However, this doesn't mean that you put your kids through a carnivore diet. Just make sure that they get sufficient animal-based protein in their early and latter stages of their growth.

With all we've discussed in mind, let's put it all into actionable form by preparing various recipes that you can prepare at home to get started on the carnivore diet.

Breakfast

Breakfast Bacon and Eggs

Serves 1

Ingredients

Pepper, freshly ground

Coarse salt

1 tablespoon unsalted butter

3 large eggs

Directions

1. Beat the eggs with a fork and set aside. Then melt butter over low heat in a medium non-stick skillet.

2. Add in the beaten egg mixture and pull them to the center of the pan using a flexible spatula.

3. Allow the liquids to run under the perimeter then cook for about 2-3 minutes or until set. Ensure you continuously move the eggs with a spatula.

4. Once done, season with pepper and salt. Serve and enjoy.

Crisp Ham and Egg Cups

Serves 2-4

Ingredients

Salt and pepper, to taste

4 large eggs

4 slices Virginia ham or black forest

Cooking spray, nonstick

Optional: fresh parsley, basil or scallions

Directions:

1. Preheat oven to about 400 deg. F. Meanwhile, use a non-stick cooking spray to lightly coat 4 muffin cups.

2. In each muffin cup, fit a slice of ham and crack an egg in each cup.

3. Now bake the ingredients in the middle oven until the egg yolks are cooked but the egg yolks still runny. This should take around 13 minutes.

4. Then you can season the eggs with salt and pepper and carefully remove the egg cups.

5. Sprinkle the dish with chopped parsley, scallions or with basil.

Sausage and Eggs

Serves 4

Ingredients

4 large eggs

1/2 teaspoon black pepper

2 tablespoons butter

1/2 teaspoon sea salt

1/2 teaspoon rosemary, dried

1/2 teaspoon thyme, dried

1 teaspoon sage, dried

1 tablespoon sweetener

1/4 pound beef liver, ground

1/2 pound beef, ground

3/4 pound pork, ground

Directions

1. In a large bowl, mix together the beef, pork, liver, salt, pepper, monk fruit, salt, seasonings and pepper.

2. Combine together using your hands until well blended, and then form the mixture into 2-inch round patties.

3. In a skillet, heat half of the oil until hot and then cook the patties for a few minutes, or until browned and cooked through.

4. Then remove the sausages from heat, add in the remaining 1 tablespoon of oil and now fry the eggs until cooked through.

5. Serve the dish with the sausages.

Quick and Easy Egg Cups

Serves 3

Ingredients

Salt and pepper

6 large eggs

3 oz. bacon, in slices

Thinly sliced fresh basil

¾ cup cheddar cheese, shredded

Directions

1. Heat your oven to 400 degrees F. Meanwhile, spray 6 muffin pans with cooking spray, non-stick.

2. Put a slice of bacon slice in each of the spray-coated pans, to form a bowl shape.

3. Sprinkle 2 tablespoons of cheddar cheese into each muffin cups if you like using cheese. Then crack one egg in each muffin cup and season with some pepper and salt.

4. At this point, bake until the egg whites are just set or for 12 to 24 minutes.

5. Serve the egg cups with basil as garnish, if you like it.

Cheese Omelet

Serves 2

Ingredients

7 oz. shredded cheddar cheese

6 eggs

3 oz. butter

Salt and pepper to taste

Directions

1. Whisk the eggs to obtain a smooth and frothy consistency.

2. Then mix in half of the cheese and season with salt and pepper.

3. In a hot frying pan, melt some butter and then pour in the cheese and egg mixture. Let the contents settle for a couple of minutes.

4. Reduce the heat and then cook until the mixture is well cooked.

5. Add in the rest of the cheese and fold. Serve while hot.

Cloud Eggs

Serves 4

Ingredients

1/2 pounds deli ham, chopped

1 cup Parmesan, freshly grated

Black pepper, freshly ground

Kosher salt

8 large eggs

Fresh chives, finely chopped for garnish

Directions

1. First preheat your oven to 450 degrees F and then line a baking sheet using a parchment paper.

2. Now separate the egg yolks from the whites, and put the yolks in a small bowl and egg whites in a large bowl.

3. Season the whites with some pepper and salt. Then whisk the egg whites using a hand mixer or a whisk. Beat until stiff peaks are well formed.

4. Now fold in the cheese, ham and the chives. Make four mounds of egg whites on a

baking sheet and then indent the centers of each to resemble nests.

5. Then bake the mounds for around 3 minutes, or until somehow golden.

6. At this point, add an egg yolk in the middle of egg white cloud. Season with pepper and salt and then bake for about 3 minutes. Once the egg yolks are set, serve.

Lunches

Easy Buffalo Wings

Serves 2

Ingredients

2 tablespoons butter

1/2 cup Frank's Red Hot Sauce

6 chicken wings

Paprika

Garlic powder

Pepper

Salt

Cayenne (optional)

Directions

1. Break the chicken meat into two pieces, the drumetets and wingettes while discarding the tips.

2. Pour a little amount of hot sauce over the meat, to lightly coat them.

2. Now season the wings and toss to coat. Turn the broiler to high and put the meat on

the oven rack, about 6 inches from the broiler.

3. Line a baking sheet using aluminum foil and then lay the wings while allowing enough space between them for easy roasting.

4. Bake for about 15 minutes then serve.

Chili Roasted Chicken Thighs

Serves: 4

Ingredients

1 tablespoon chili powder

2 pounds boneless chicken thighs

Lime wedges for serving, optional

Fresh cilantro for garnish

Directions

1. First heat the oven to 375 degrees F.

2. To a sheet pan, add in the chicken and then drizzle the meat with olive oil. Turn it around to coat in oil.

2. Season the chicken with salt, chili powder and pepper and now roast the chicken for 15 minutes.

3. Once cooked through, remove the meat from the heat and sprinkle with cilantro. Serve with lime wedges if you like.

Easy Mahi Mahi

Servings 4

Ingredients

1 teaspoon salt

1 tablespoon Herbes de Provence

1/2 cup butter melted

4 Mahi Mahi filets

Directions

1. First heat your oven to 375 degrees F. Meanwhile, put the mahi mahi fillets in a 9 by 13 inch pan.

2. Pour melted butter over the fillets and season with salt and Herbes de Provence.

3. Bake in the preheated oven for about 20 minutes, and then remove from heat. Let cool for 5 minutes and serve.

Spicy Baked Chicken

Servings 3

Ingredients

1 pound boneless, skinless chicken breasts

1/4 teaspoon black pepper freshly ground

1/2 teaspoon sea salt

1/2 cup mild or spicy salsa

4 ounces cream cheese cut into large chunks

1 teaspoon finely chopped parsley

Directions

1. First heat your oven to 350 degrees F. Then add the salsa and cream cheese to a heavy-weight cooking pan.

2. Put the saucepan over low heat and cook, stirring now and again until the cheese melts and fully blends with the salsa. Season with salt and pepper and remove the mixture from heat.

3. Layer the skinless meat on a prepared baking dish and add in the cheese and salsa mixture on top, to fully cover the breast.

4. Now bake the mixture until the center of the chicken meat indicates 180 degrees on

the meat thermometer, or for about 40 to 45 minutes.

5. Take out of the oven and top with fresh parsley if you like it. You can serve immediately or keep the chicken in the fridge in freezer bags.

6. Be aware that cooked chicken meat may hardly last beyond a week even when frozen.

Pressure-Cooker Octopus

Serves 6

Ingredients

2 1/2-pound whole octopus, rinsed well

Sea salt

Directions

1. Put the octopus in the cooking pot and add sufficient amount of water to cover the fish.

2. Add large pinches of salt and seal the instant pot. Cook at high pressure for approximately 15 minutes.

3. Then quick release to depressurize the instant pot. Slide a paring knife into the thickest part of the octopus tentacles to check if the octopus is tender. If so, it should slide easily.

4. In case the octopus isn't tender, cook for another 5 minutes. Allow the fish to cool inside the cooking liquid and then drain.

5. To serve, cut out and discard the hard beak found in the center of the base of its body where its tentacles converge.

6. Cut out the section of the head with eyes and discard, and separate the tentacles into

individual pieces. These and the other parts
are edible.

7. Serve the octopus cold. Just cut the head
into pieces and the tentacles too then add it
to a salad or other meal and enjoy.

Instant Pot Steamed Crab Legs

Servings: 4

Ingredients

4 tablespoons butter, melted

¾ cup water

Lemon juice

2 lbs. frozen crab legs

Directions

1. Place the steamer basket into the instant pot then put the crab legs on it.

2. Add in water and lock the lid in place.

3. Then cook for 2 minutes on high pressure then quick release. The crab meat, once cooked, should be bright pink in color.

4. Combine juice with some melted butter then serve.

Dinner

Spice-Rubbed Bison Tenderloin

Serves: 4

Ingredients

4 six-ounce bison or beef tenderloin filets

½ teaspoon gray sea salt or pink rock salt

1 teaspoon minced fresh ginger root

½ teaspoon allspice

2 teaspoon cumin seeds, dry-toasted and ground

2 teaspoon coriander seeds, ground

1 teaspoon cinnamon

2 tablespoon minced garlic

2 sprigs fresh rosemary

Directions

1. Mix together ginger root, spices, garlic and rosemary in a small bowl and set aside.

2. Put the bison or beef on a 12 x 12 inch glass baking dish, and then coat both sides using the spice mix.

3. Now preheat the broiler on low and then put the fillets under it, around 6 inches from heat. Use medium low heat if using a grill pan on a stove.

4. Drizzle the meat with broth or filtered water to keep it moist. This also ensures your spices don't catch fire.

5. Grill or broil for around 4 to 6 minutes until done, while checking the meat not to overcook it.

6. As soon as it is done, remove from the grill or oven and allow cool. Serve and enjoy.

Mesquite Garlic Trout

Serves 4

Ingredients

4 tablespoons minced garlic

1 teaspoon salt

1 teaspoon mesquite seasoning

2 pounds trout

Directions

1. First heat your outside grill or oven to 450 degrees F. Meanwhile, cut the tail and head of a gutted and the well cleaned fish.

2. Put 4 to 5 tablespoons of minced garlic in the open belly of the fish.

3. Pour some salt and mesquite seasoning on the garlic and then wait for the trout belly to close.

4. Put the fish on an aluminum foil and loosely wrap it on the fish to fully seal it but with some air spaces.

5. Put the trout on the grill or oven and now cook for about 20 minutes. As soon as the meat can easily flake, stop cooking and serve.

Easy Slow Cooker Taco Meat

Serves 4-6

Ingredients

2 lbs. ground beef

Spices

1/4 teaspoon crushed red pepper

1/4 teaspoon paprika

1/2 teaspoon onion powder

1/2 teaspoon garlic powder

1/2 teaspoon dried oregano

1/2 teaspoon coriander

1 teaspoon black pepper

1 teaspoon sea salt

1 teaspoon cumin

1 tablespoon chili powder

3 tablespoons tomato paste

Directions

1. Mix together all the spices in a small bowl.

2. Add the spices, tomato paste and the beef to the crock-pot. Mix together using a spoon.

3. Cook on low heat for 4 hours, and then break u the meat using a spoon.

4. Remove the meat from the crock-pot using a slotted spoon.

Cheese Stuffed Bacon Cheeseburger

Serves 2

Ingredients

1 tablespoon butter

1 teaspoon Cajun seasoning

1/2 teaspoon pepper

1 teaspoon salt

2 oz. cheddar cheese

1 oz. mozzarella cheese

2 slices bacon, pre-cooked

8 oz. ground beef

Directions

1. Use all spices to season the ground beef and mix together lightly.

2. Cube the mozzarella cheese and slice the cheddar.

3. Now grab the seasoned ground beef, and make rough patties from it. Once done, put the mozzarella inside and now enclose the cheese with the beef.

4. In a pan, heat a tablespoon of butter until bubbling and hot. Add one burger to the hot pan.

5. Cover using a cloche and cook for 2-3 minutes.

6. Then flip the burger and put the cheddar on top. Cover the pan with cloche again and cook for 1-2 minutes.

7. Finally chop bacon slice in half and put it over the burger. Serve.

Cheesy Bacon Chicken

Serves: 6

Ingredients

4 ounce shredded cheddar

1/2 pound bacon, cut strips in half

2 tablespoons seasoning rub

5-6 chicken breasts, cut in half width wise

Barbecue sauce, optional

Directions

1. Heat the oven to 400 degrees F. Meanwhile, coat a baking sheet that is rimmed with cooking spray.

2. With the season rub, season both sides of chicken and top each breast with bacon.

3. Bake the chicken until it looks crispy and the meat thermometer indicates 160 degrees, or for approximately 30 minutes.

4. Then remove from the hot oven and distribute the cheese over bacon strips. Return to the oven and now bake until the cheese is bubbly and golden, or for another 10 minutes.

5. Serve the cheesy bacon chicken with barbeque sauce if you like.

Low Carb Skillet Lasagna

Serves 4

Ingredients

1 teaspoon fresh oregano, chopped

1 cup shredded mozzarella cheese divided, about 4 ounces

4 slices thin roast chicken breast from deli counter

24 ounce jar no sugar added marinara sauce

2 teaspoons fine sea salt

1 pound 80% lean ground beef

Directions

1. Brown the beef in a 10 inch cast iron skillet over medium high heat, while seasoning the meat with sea salt as it cooks.

2. Cook the beef for around 5 minutes or until cooked through. Keep breaking up the beef using a spatula as it cooks.

2. Add in the sauce, stir to blend then push half of the cooked beef off one side of the skillet.

3. Now put a layer of sliced chicken breast on the bottom of the cooking pan and top the meat with half cup of shredded cheese.

4. Then scoop the beef on top of left over bacon to create an even layer. Top with the reserved 1/2 cup of cheese and sprinkle with some oregano.

5. Cover the mixture and heat on low to fully melt the cheese.

Snacks And Appetizers

Lemon Garlic Chicken Skewers

Serves 8

Ingredients

2 tablespoon fresh parsley, chopped

3/4 cup Tessemae's Lemon Garlic

4 chicken breasts, cut into 1 inch cubes

Directions

1. To a bowl or zip lock bag, add the lemon garlic dressing and chicken and let coat for a few minutes. Keep it chilled for 1 to 3 hours.

2. Meanwhile, preheat the grill to around 500 degrees F and then start treading the chicken onto the skewers. If using wooden skewers, soak them in water about 30 minutes before use.

3. Once the grill is hot enough, put the skewers on the grill and cook until the chicken is well cooked, while flipping halfway through to enable even cooking.

4. After about 15 minutes or so, remove from the grill and garnish with fresh herbs such as parsley or others.

5. You can also cook the chicken under a broiler or a grill pan and ensure the internal temperature reaches 160 degrees before serving.

Tortilla Pork Rind Wraps

Yield: 8 wraps

Serving Size: 1 wrap

Ingredients

1/4 teaspoon ground cumin

1/2 teaspoon garlic powder

3 ounces pork rinds, crushed

4 large eggs

Butter

Directions

1. Mix together eggs, garlic powder, pork rinds and cumin in a food processor or blender until well combined and smooth.

2. Add about ¼ cups of water, and continue blending; and add more water as required to achieve pancake batter consistency.

3. Now over medium-low heat, melt half teaspoon of coconut or avocado oil in a non-stick skillet.

4. Swirl to coat the pan, and then add around 3 tablespoons of batter. Spread it

thinly over the pan using a rubber spatula, almost to edges.

5.   Cook the batter until the bottom starts to brown, or for approximately 1 minute.

6.   With a spoon, carefully loosen the edges and flip the pancake. Cook the other side for approximately 1 minute.

7. Repeat steps 2 and 3 with the rest of the batter, but only add oil to the skillet if required. You need less oil in the pan to easily spread batter.

8. Continue adding water to the batter as required throughout cooking as it may thicken with time.

9. Serve when done with the cooking.

Slow-Cooker Garlicky Shrimp

Serves: 6

Ingredients

1 tablespoon flat-leaf parsley, minced

2 pounds extra-large raw shrimp, peeled and deveined

1/4 teaspoon crushed red pepper flakes

1/4 teaspoon black pepper, freshly ground

1 teaspoon kosher salt

1 teaspoon smoked Spanish paprika

6 cloves garlic, thinly sliced

3/4 cup melted butter

Directions

1. Mix together crushed pepper flakes, black pepper, salt, paprika, garlic and oil in a crockpot. Stir the mixture to incorporate.

2. Then cover and cook for 30 minutes on high heat settings. Now stir in shrimp to coat it then cover and cook for another 10 minutes.

3. Stir to help the shrimp cook evenly until all of the fish meat is opaque or for about 10 minutes or so.

4. Move the fish and its sauce to a serving dish then sprinkles with parsley to garnish. Serve it warm.

Homemade Greek Yogurt

Serves: 4

Ingredients

½ cup plain full-fat yogurt

½ gallon whole milk

Directions

1. To make Greek yoghurt, line a fine mesh using 3 layers of cheesecloth, then put it in a large bowl.

2. Move the yoghurt to a sieve and allow the liquid whey to drain so that you can get preferred yoghurt consistency. This should take around 4 hours.

3. Chill the yoghurt and then serve.

Salmon and Cream Cheese Bites

Serves 4

Ingredients

50 grams cream cheese

1 teaspoon dried dill

50 g fresh or smoked salmon slices

50 g shredded/grated cheese

1/2 teaspoon salt

250 ml cow/goat milk

6 medium sized eggs

Directions

1. In a large pouring jug, whisk together eggs, coconut milk and salt and then fold in dill, smoked salmon, grated cheese and chopped cream cheese.

2. Pour the batter into greased silicon molds or mini muffin trays. Bake the mixture at about 180 degrees C for about 10 to 15 minutes.

3. Allow to cool and then serve.

Low Carb Slow Cooker Cheesecake

Serves 8

Ingredients

1/2 tablespoon vanilla

1 cup splenda or other no-calorie sweetener

3 eggs

3 -8 oz. packages cream cheese

Directions

1. Allow the cream cheese to come to warm up then put it in a large bowl. Add in a sweetener.

2. Using a mixer, combine cream cheese and the sweetener until well incorporated.

3. Then add in eggs one by one, and mix to blend. Now coat the slow cooker bowl with cooking spray and then pour the cream cheese.

4. Add a few cups of water to the slow cooker to last for 2 hours and then put the cheesecake into the cooking bowl.

5. Close the lid in place and cook on high heat for about 2 to 2 and a half hours.

6. If the mixture puff up at any time of the cooking, let cooking progress for about 2 hours. Cook until a knife inserted in the mixture comes out clean.

Conclusion

We have come to the end of the book. Thank you for reading and congratulations for reading until the end.

Adopting the carnivore diet is the best thing you will ever do for your health. There are astonishing amount of benefits to your health, and plenty of research to back it up. Just as with any other standard low carb diets, the carnivore diet will cause a profound shift in the body and brain chemistry rather swiftly. Embrace these changes because they are always positive and healthy.

If you found the book valuable, can you recommend it to others? One way to do that is to post a review on Amazon.

Click here to leave a review for this book on Amazon!

Thank you and good luck!